A PLANT WONDER DRUG?

The vine called Cat's Claw is reputed to improve immune function, relieve arthritis and prostate problems—even to have cured cases of cancer. In Oriental and South American healing traditions, it is used to treat abscesses, asthma, fever, ulcers, rheumatism, wounds and many other conditions. But myth and mystery distort the facts about the "wonder drug," and Alexander Schauss has searched out the remarkable truth about what Cat's Claw can do, how it does it, and how you can experience the benefits of this unique and potent herb.

ABOUT THE AUTHOR

Alexander Schauss, Ph.D., a research psychologist and mental health therapist, holds associate professorships at colleges of naturopathic medicine in Oregon and Arizona, and is Research Director of the American Institute for Biosocial Research's Life Sciences Division. Dr. Schauss has spent more than 20 years studying the relationships between diet, nutrition, brain function and behavior, and has held various positions in social service and criminal justice agencies as well as in academic institutions. He is author or coauthor of more than 50 publications, including the Good Health Guides *Nutrition and Behavior* and *Anorexia and Bulimia,* and has presented papers on the nutrition-behavior link at many American and international conferences.

The Health Benefits of Cat's Claw

Its role in treating cancer, arthritis, prostate problems, asthma and many other chronic conditions

Alexander Schauss, Ph.D.
author of *Nutrition and Behavior*

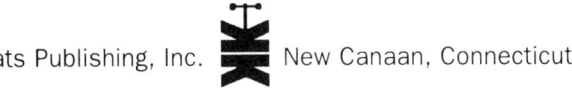

Keats Publishing, Inc.   New Canaan, Connecticut

The Health Benefits of Cat's Claw is intended solely for informational and educational purposes, and not as medical advice. Please consult a medical or health professional if you have questions about your health.

THE HEALTH BENEFITS OF CAT'S CLAW
Copyright © 1996 by Alexander Schauss
All Rights Reserved

No part of this book may be reproduced in any form without the written consent of the publisher.

ISBN: 0-87983-757-8

Printed in the United States of America

Keats Good Health Guides are published by
Keats Publishing, Inc.
27 Pine Street (Box 876)
New Canaan, Connecticut 06840-0876

Contents

	Pages
Introduction	7
Recent Interest in Cat's Claw	11
The Botany of Cat's Claw	14
Uncaria in Traditional Medicine	15
Peruvian Barks	26
Uncaria Tomentosa (Wild.) DC—"Cat's Claw"	29
Ecological Issues	37
Toxicology	37
How to Be Sure It's Genuine Cat's Claw	39
References	45

INTRODUCTION

In recent years there has been considerable medical interest in the bark, root and leaves of a vine found in Peru, Columbia, Ecuador and other Latin American countries, called Cat's Claw—the botanical name is *Uncaria tomentosa*.

The Spanish call this vine "Uña de Gato," which translates to English as "cat's claw." In the eastern Andes Mountains of Peru, this vine can grow to over 26 meters in length and at its base be as thick as a watermelon.

The botanical name of the genus of this species, *Uncaria*, comes from the Latin word *uncus*, meaning hook, as these plants bear on their stems\strong, downward-curving hooks. These hooks enable the vine to climb trees and other vegetation. The hooks resemble a cat's claw.

Numerous anecdotes have been reported in recent years that hail Cat's Claw as the "wonder drug of the botanical kingdom." Consumers who have benefited from using Cat's Claw have claimed it has improved their immune function, resolved their arthritis, cured them of prostate problems, and even cured them of benign and malignant tumors. Is the excitement justified?

I first heard about Cat's Claw in 1985. But it wasn't until four years later that I heard so many reports of Cat's Claw's benefits that I attempted to contact an old acquaintance at the Peruvian Ministry of Health in Lima.

Since Peru is the world's primary commercial source for the bark and root of Cat's Claw, I hoped that my Peruvian friend could send me whatever research his government had collected on this vine. That effort and several years of accumulated papers on Cat's Claw, combined with increasing promotion of this vine, compelled me to write this book. Not just because I thought the subject might be of interest to others, but because I had heard so much misinformation being promoted about this fascinating botanical medicine.

Cat's Claw Fact and Fancy

Here is just a small sample of the type of misinformation about Cat's Claw I came across:

Claim: "You can only find Cat's Claw in Peru."
Fact: Cat's Claw is found throughout Central and South America, in swamps and at high altitudes. Wherever growing conditions are conducive to its survival. The major *commercial* source of Cat's Claw products is Peru. However, it grows in abundance in other areas of Latin America. In banana-growing regions along the Atlantic coast, Cat's Claw is considered a nuisance weed. In each banana-producing country it is called by a different local name.

Claim: "Only the inner bark is therapeutic."
Fact: From pre-Columbians to modern native healers, virtually every part of the plant has been found to be of medicinal value, including the root, hook, leaf, and bark. Higher levels of certain vital therapeutic compounds (alkaloids) are found in the root, not the bark. However, the bark contains some substances that may be therapeutic that are not found in the root. The levels of the therapeutic compounds in the root, bark and leaf can vary significantly, explaining why it is important to buy Cat's Claw products from reliable manufacturers who always test *each* lot for key constituents (especially several of the oxindole alkaloids).

Claim: "It is illegal to export the root of Cat's Claw from Peru."
Fact: Peru has no law that prohibits the export of Cat's Claw root. However, it does ban the exportation of *any* whole plant without government approval.

Claim: "Cat's Claw is completely safe."
Fact: False. The dosage, form of preparation, etc., varies. For example, although the therapeutic dose may be 20 grams

per day (in spaced dosages), one may have to begin by taking no more than 2 to 3 grams per day at first and gradually increase the dosage until reaching the therapeutic dose in several weeks. Otherwise constipation may not be the only problem encountered. Also, there is insufficient evidence that Cat's Claw is safe in pregnancy. In fact, one of its traditional uses is as an abortifacient (a substance that can induce an abortion).

Claim: "If the herb is adequate in the alkaloid isopteropodine, it is genuine Cat's Claw."

Fact: Simply testing for one of 14 alkaloids in Cat's Claw is inadequate evidence that it is the genuine product. To be really sure, several constituents known to be found in Cat's Claw need to be analytically identified by an *independent* laboratory.

Obviously, as can be seen from these examples, it is important to separate fact from fiction. In recent years, the growing consumer and trade interest in Cat's Claw has come from a number of newspaper and magazine articles that have touted the "wondrous" properties of the "miracle vine" from Peru. What is confusing is how often the articles mix drug development research outcome reports with botanical research.

Many of these articles have also claimed that native Peruvians brew a tea from the bark or root of Cat's Claw to treat everything from rheumatoid diseases to tumors, the same way their pre-Columbian ancestors did hundreds of years ago. However, this is true of only a very small number of Peruvians. Studies that have scientifically demonstrated a beneficial effect against certain cancers have been conducted by drug development researchers investigating isolated chemical compounds found in Cat's Claw. In one paragraph they are talking about drug research, while in the next paragraph they are discussing traditional usage. There is a difference! Taking a drug and drinking a decoction (especially a prepared brew or a soaked part of the plant) are very different.

Reported Benefits

None of these concerns, however, discredit the benefits consumers claim they have derived from taking Cat's Claw to treat their malady. It is not uncommon to hear a cancer patient in Peru describe how he visited a local healer and was given a decoction of Cat's Claw for several days or weeks to treat a tumor. Adding to the interest are intriguing reports from pharmaceutical researchers who have been studying the properties of Cat's Claw by identifying the vine's potentially therapeutic compounds. For example, one study demonstrated that an isolated constituent in Cat's Claw enhanced cytostatic action in animals, resulting in a suppression in the rate of proliferation of cancerous cells. Another study demonstrated that similar constituents in the plant increased phagocytic—cell-devouring—action, an immune activity important to patients infected with viruses or the infamous retrovirus, HIV, that contributes to AIDS.

These reports have increased the level of commercial interest in Cat's Claw to a remarkable level. One distributor of Claw's Claw root in the United States reported that sales of his product increased tenfold in just one year!

By 1996, more than 50 dietary supplement manufacturers in the United States were offering various Cat's Claw products to consumers. And sales were brisk. In response, the Peruvian government was even considering restricting the amount of Cat's Claw leaving Peru to insure that an adequate supply would always be available for future generations.

The export of Cat's Claw root and bark has provided the Peruvian government with many jobs for natives living in remote areas of the country, while contributing millions of dollars to its treasury from an inpouring of foreign currencies.

RECENT INTEREST IN CAT'S CLAW

Although the scientific and commercial interest in Cat's Claw can be traced back at least a quarter of a century, the real beginning to our modern appreciation for this vine needs to be credited to a German-born researcher, Arturo Brell.

One account of Brell's history is particularly informative in understanding how Cat's Claw became well known to many[1]:

> Born Arthur Brell in Upper Bavaria, in 1904, he studied Natural Sciences in Munich (Germany). However, the young Brell dreamt of the exotic Americas of the Aztecs and Incas. It was not until a chance meeting that turned his dreams into reality. A cleric called Schaffer, then leader and parish priest of a group of German colonists in Pozuzo, suggested he make the trip to Peru to set up a school with the aim of educating the region's natives in the ways of the Western world.
>
> Three years after his arrival, Brell had become a prosperous coffee grower in Chanchamayo. It was there, living side by side with the Campa and Amuesha Indians, that he was able to become familiar with the area's tribal customs. Among other things, he noted that the locals, despite living among the constant smoke of cooking fires and broiling most of their food over charcoal, both factors exposing them to a daily absorption of the carcinogenic elements found in tar, were untroubled by cancer. Years of painstaking research led him to the conclusion that this state of affairs had to do fundamentally with a powerful immunological system. Brell himself, having already obtained Uncaria extracts, had eliminated his long-standing rheumatic complaints, and noticed that his complexion had improved and his hair had grown rapidly.

The day of reckoning came when another colonist, his friend Schuler, finding himself helpless against a terminal case of lung cancer, went to him for help. To the incredulity and amazement of the doctors who had been treating him, after a couple of years of dosing him with preparations made from the miraculous plant, the sick man made a full recovery. Until the day he died (from other causes) at eighty-eight years of age, the old man went to working, in the company of his children, in his tropical sawmill in Villa Rica and, according to those who knew him, even occasionally smoking a cigarette made from his own tobacco. In August 1974, Schuler wrote a letter of gratitude to Arturo Brell, saying: "If it hadn't been for your treatment and herb extracts I wouldn't be alive today, four years after being diagnosed with terminal illness by the doctors."

Arturo Brell died in Lima, Peru, in 1978. Before he died, Brell began to hear from enough researchers curious about his "miraculous" plant, to assure him that his long-standing study of Cat's Claw would continue well past his death.

It also did not hurt that several noted Latin American actors and industrialists claimed that Cat's Claw cured them of their cancers. Dominican TV soap actor Andrés Garcia told the press he completely recovered from prostate cancer thanks to Cat's Claw. Shortly thereafter, Manuel Moreyra Loredo, former director of the Central Reserve Bank of Peru, told a New York radio audience that his cure from several malignant tumors in his lungs and brain was due to Cat's Claw.

In the early 1970s, at the urging of Brell and others, and at the prompting of then President Richard Nixon, the U.S. National Cancer Institute initiated *in vitro* (test tube) cell studies of the bark and root of *Uncaria tomentosa*. Although the results with certain leukemia cells were promising, all research on the extract of the plant unexpectedly stopped the following year. Repeated attempts to revive further interest in Cat's Claw failed.

At about the same time, the Peruvian National Institute of Neoplastic Diseases began studying the plant's anticancer qualities. But eventually enthusiasm and funding to support this effort waned as it became increasingly evident that the whole root or bark of Cat's Claw might be more effective than any one particular compound found in the plant. This lessened pharmaceutical interest, since a whole plant can not be patent-protected. Nevertheless, several Peruvian universities continued to study and publish information on the plant's phytomedicinal properties.

In Europe, a self-educated ethnologist and ethnobotanist, Klaus Keplinger, organized the first clinical trials on humans, despite limited funds. But unlike Peruvian studies, Keplinger's interest was in isolating compounds found in the root or bark of Cat's Claw that could be patented. One has therefore to be very careful when reviewing the literature on the therapeutic benefits of Cat's Claw not to confuse reports from Keplinger's lab with claims made by native healers.

As consumer demand for Cat's Claw has increased, so has the need for impartial information about the product. So let me begin this discussion by saying my interest in Cat's Claw is simple: to raise, and do my best to answer, some basic questions. Here are some of them:

- Does Cat's Claw really do what some claim, or is the excitement premature?
- Do consumers know how much Cat's Claw to take? Do they know how to prepare the root or bark?
- What is the effective dosage range? How long does it take to reach this effective dose while avoiding common side effects?
- Can taking too much be toxic? Is it safe to take with another drug or drugs?
- Which part of the plant is more therapeutic, the root or the bark?
- How can we be sure that the product we buy is genuine Cat's Claw?

THE BOTANY OF CAT'S CLAW

Some background on the botany of Cat's Claw is in order to help us understand its unique chemistry.

Uncaria tomentosa (Cat's Claw) is one of 34 species of the genus *Uncaria*, which is a member of the order Rubiaceae. This family of plants has a number of interesting similarities in chemical structure, which provide us insights into why the genus, including *U. tomentosa*, possesses medicinal qualities.

The Genus Uncaria

The genus *Uncaria* is found in tropical and subtropical regions of Central and South America, Africa and Asia. No species of *Uncaria* has been found in North America (other than southern Mexico), Australia, New Zealand or Europe.

Table 1 lists the 34 known species of the genus *Uncaria* (family Rubiaceae) that have been identified worldwide. The Rubiaceae family is comprised of some 6,000 to 7,000 species distributed among some 500 genera that inhabit primarily tropical and moist environments around the world. The common bond between the various genera of the Rubiaceae is their precursor chemical, secologanin. The combination of secologanin with either tryptamine or tryptophan results in two chemicals, strictosidine or carboxystrictosidine, which are the precursors of the indole and quinoline alkaloids. It is these alkaloids that are of therapeutic interest to phytochemists and medical researchers studying *Uncaria* and other genera in the family Rubiaceae.

UNCARIA IN TRADITIONAL MEDICINE

The many species of the genus *Uncaria* found around the world, listed in Table 1, have a long history of use in Chinese, Taiwanese, Japanese, Malaysian and Central and South American traditional medicine.

Table 1

SPECIES OF THE *UNCARIA* GENUS (FAMILY RUBIACEAE)

Uncaria acuivata Wild. (occurs only in the Guyanas)
Uncaria attenuata Korth
Uncaria bernaysii F.v.Muell (occurs only in New Guinea)
Uncaria bulusanensis (Elm.) Rids. msc.
Uncaria callophylla Bl. ex Korth
Uncaria dasyoneura Korth
Uncaria elliptica
Uncaria ferrea D.C.
Uncaria florida Vidal
Uncaria formosana (Mats.) Hayata
Uncaria gambir (Hunt) Roxb. (also *U. gambier*)
Uncaria gambir Thw.
Uncaria guianensis (Aubl.) Gmel.
Uncaria hirsuta Haviland
Uncaria homomalla Miq.
Uncaria kawakamii Hayata
Uncaria laevigata Wall. ex G. Don
Uncaria lancifolia Hutch.
Uncaria lanosa
Uncaria longiflora (Poir.) Merr.
Uncaria macrophylla Wallich
Uncaria orientalis Guill
Uncaria pteropoda
Uncaria quadrangularis
Uncaria rhynchophylla (Miq.) Jackson
Uncaria rostrata Pierre ex Pitrard
Uncaria salaccensis
Uncaria scandens (J.E. Smith) Hutch.
Uncaria sessilifructus (Roxb.)
Uncaria sinensis Oliver
Uncaria thwaitesii
Uncaria tomentosa (Wild) DC
Uncaria tonkinensis

In traditional Peruvian medicine, *U. tomentosa* has been used for a variety of ailments and applications:

Abscesses	Hemorrhage
Arthritis	Inflammation
Asthma	Menstrual irregularity
Cancer	Rheumatism
Contraception	Skin disorders
Fever	Urinary tract infections
Gastric ulcer	Wounds
Growing (bone) pains	

In traditional Chinese medicine, five species of the genus *Uncaria* (*U. hirsuta, U. macrophylla, U. rhynchopylla, U. sessilifructus*, and *U. slnensis*) are known collectively by their Chinese name, *gou-teng*; the botanical name for this plant is *Ramulus uncariae cum uncis*. The practitioners of traditional Chinese medicine use primarily the stems and hooks of the plant to prepare an oral decoction to treat such conditions as: headache, vertigo (dizziness) due to hypertension, convulsions with high fever, irritability, and nervousness.[2] There is no reference in traditional Chinese medical texts to the use of *Uncaria* for the treatment of auto-immune disorders, immune deficiencies, tumors or cancer.

The earliest known reference to any of the five species of *Uncaria* in traditional Chinese medicine is found in *The Origins of the Materia Medica* written by Li Zhong-Li during the Ming Dynasty. This suggests that the use of *Uncaria* in traditional Chinese medicine has existed for more than 500 years.[3] Of the five species of *Uncaria*, the most important species used in traditional Chinese medicine are *U. rhynchophylla* and *U. gambir*.[4,5] These two species are recommended most often in traditional Chinese texts.

In Taiwanese folk medicine (Thang-kau-tin), *U. rhynchophylla* and *U. hirsuta* are used in the treatment of arthritis[6] and hepatitis[7], and as anti-inflammatory and liver-protective agents.[8] Studies have demonstrated that these species of *Uncaria* are capable of suppressing free radical damage, giving further support to the theory that *Uncaria* species are active oxygen scavengers against the tissue injury caused by superoxide radicals and/or hydroxyl radicals.[9] Superoxide radicals and hydroxyl radicals have been implicated in the inflammatory process associated with rheumatoid arthritis. Clinical studies have shown that oxygen scavengers such as vitamin E and superoxide dismutase are capable of alleviating inflammation in rheumatoid arthritis.

Healers in the Malaysian peninsula, including Malaysia, Thailand and Burma, also have a long history of the use of *Uncaria* in their traditional curative systems. In 1930 a paper was published describing several species of *Uncaria* that are found in the Malaysian peninsula and used to treat wounds, fever, headache, bacterial infections, febrile convulsions, epigastric disturbances, ulcers, gastrointestinal discomforts and fungal infections. For example, in the area now known as the "Golden Triangle" of Thailand, traditional healers prepare a decoction of the root of two local *Uncaria* species to treat bladder stones, various urinary problems, and as a diuretic.[11]

In South America, there is also a long traditional history of use. It is estimated that two of the species of the genus *Uncaria* found only in South and Central America (including southern Mexico), *U. guianensis* and *U. tomentosa*, have been used by local healers for at least 500 years. *U. guianensis* is said to be used in traditional South American medicine as a treatment for wound healing and intestinal ailments.[12]

Ethnobotanical studies have found reference to the use of *Uncaria* among many traditional healers in Costa Rica, Colombia, Brazil, Ecuador and Peru.[13] Unfortunately, sometimes the two species are referred to by their Spanish name, *uña de gato*, causing some concern within the domestic and international herbal marketplace as to which species is being sold. Local herbalists in those South American countries can generally differentiate the species by their color. But color can be deceiving. It doesn't take much effort to add certain powdered barks from other trees or shrubs to give a product just the right color. Consumers are advised to make sure that what they are getting is real Cat's Claw. At the end of this book I have listed several reliable sources of genuine Cat's Claw.

What are the active constituents in *Uncaria* that have promoted hundreds of years of use? What are the common chemicals in *Uncaria* that give rise to its use by traditional healers in Asia and South America?

ALKALOIDS FOUND IN *UNCARIA*

Alkaloids are nitrogen-based substances found in plants. They are usually bitter. Most alkaloids have pharmacological activity. Examples of some common alkaloids that most people know of are atropine, caffeine, morphine, nicotine, quinine and strychnine.

The indole alkaloids comprise the second largest single group of plant-based chemicals known. Many alkaloids are particularly valued for their medicinal effect. For example, the tranquilizer reserpine is an alkaloid that is found in *Rauwolfia serpentina* and used for the treatment of high blood pressure. The legendary aphrodisiac yohimbine is found in the bark of *Pausinystalia yohimbe*. This same alkaloid is also used as an antidepressant. The Madagascar periwinkle (*Vinca rosea*) contains over 60 alkaloids in its root and leaves, two of which (vinblastine and vincristine) are useful in the treatment of leukemia.

Analytical studies of several hundred samples of the 34 known species of *Uncaria* have resulted in the identification of over 50 alkaloids. Many of these alkaloids have known therapeutic value and will be discussed later. Those alkaloids that have been analytically identified in various species of *Uncaria* are shown in Table 2. Among many of the alkaloids found in *Uncaria*, the most interesting ones are the indole and oxindole alkaloids.

Table 2

ALKALOIDS IDENTIFIED IN *UNCARIA*

Akuammigine	Isoajmalicine	Rotundifoline
Angustine	Isocorynoxeine	Roxburghine D
Angustoline	Isodihydrocadambine	Roxburghine X
Cadambine	Isoformosanine (uncarine A)	Salacine
Carboxystrictosidine		Secorhynchophylline
Corynantheine	Isogambirdine	Speciophylline (uncarine D)
Corynoxeine	Isomitraphylline	Strictosamide
Dihydrocadambine	Isopteropodine (uncarine E)	Tetrahydroalstonine
Dihydrocorynantheine		Uncarine A
Epiajmalicine	Israuniticine	(isoformosanine)

Formosamine (uncarine B)	Isorauniticine	Uncarine A
Gambirdine	pseudoindoxyl	(isoformosanine)
(gambirtannine)	Isorhynchophylline	Uncarine B (formosamine)
Geissoschizine	Isorotundifoline	Uncarine C (pteropodine)
Harmine	Metraphylline	Uncarine D
Heteroyohimbine	Pteropodine (uncarine C)	(speciophylline)
Hirsuteine	Rauniticine	Uncarine E
Hirsutine	Rauniticine oxindole A	(isopteropodine)
Hydroalstonine	Rhynchophine	Uncarine F
Hydroxyrauniticine	Rhynchophylline	Vallesiachotamine

The alkaloids found in specific species of *Uncaria* are shown in Table 3. You will note that the types of alkaloids found in any species of *Uncaria* can vary significantly. In fact, there is no alkaloid or group of alkaloids that are found in all species of *Uncaria*.

Table 3

ALKALOIDS IDENTIFIED IN VARIOUS *UNCARIA* SPECIES

Uncaria species	*Alkaloids (non-alkaloids shown in italics)*
U. attenuata Korth	mitraphylline, isoajmalicine, uncarine B, hydroxyrauniticine, salacine, heteroyohimbine alkaloids (tetrahydroalstonine, rauniticine and isorauniticine) secorhynchophylline
U. bernaysii	angustine and heteroyohimbine
U. callophylla Bl. ex Korth	heteroyohimbine (gambirine), dihydrocorynantheine
U. elliptica R. Br. exG. Don	roxburghine D, roxburghine X, formosamine, isomitraphylline, mitraphylline, epiajmalicine, raunticine, isorauniticine, rauniticine oxindole A, hydroalstonine, isorauniticine pseudoindoxyl, isoajmalicine; *rutin and (-)-epicatechin (flavonoids)*
U. florida Vidal	pteropodine, speciophylline, and isopteropodine
U. gambir (Hunt) Roxburgh	heteroyohimbine gambirdine (also "gambirtannine") and (isogambirdine), and mitraphylline; *d-catechin, dl-catchenin, l-epicatechin, d-epicatechin, (catecholtannins) acetoxydihydronomilin (limonin triterpene); gambiriin A1, A2, A3, B1, B2, and B3 (flavonids); quercitin*

U. guianensis (Aubl.) Gmel.	angustine, rhynchophylline, isorhynchophylline, mitraphylline, dihydrocorynantheine, hirsutine and hirsuteine; *four quinovic acids*
U. homomalla Miq.	angustine and angustoline
U. kawakamii Hayata	isoformosanine, formosanine, and mitraphylline
U. pteropoda	isopteropodine, pteropodine
U. quadrangularis Geddes	mitraphylline, isomitraphylline, pteropodine and isopteropodine
U. rhynchophylla Miquel	rhynchophylline, isorhynchophylline, corynoxeine, isocorynoxeine, corynantheine, dihydrocorynantheine, hirsutine, hirsuteine, isodihydrocadambine, dihydrocadambine, cadambine, geissoschizine, akuammigine, angustine, angustoline, vallesiachotamine, strictosamide, rhynchophine, formosanan, uncarine A (isoformosanine), uncarine B (formosanine), uncarine (pteropodine), uncarine D, uncarine E (isopteropodine), uncarine F; *(-)-epicatechin (a catecholtannin), trifolin and hyperin (hyperoside) (flavonols)*
U. sinensis (Oliv.) Havil	dihydrocorynantheine, corynantheine, hirsutine, hirsuteine, geissoschizine, isodihydrocadambine, harmine, rhynchophylline, isorhynchophylline, corynoxeine, akuammigine; *mitraphyllic acid, isomitraphyllic acids (glycosides)*
U. tomentosa Wild DC	isopteropodine, pteropodine, mitraphylline, hirsuteine, isomitraphylline, rhynchophylline, isorynchophylline, hirsutine, speciophylline, dihydrocorynantheine, uncarine F, carboxystrictosidine, isorotundifoline, rotundifoline; *beta-sitosterol, stigmasterol, and campestrol (steroids), three novel polyhydroxylated triterpenes, three major glycosides and six quinovic acid glycosides (in the bark) and a seventh in the root, (--) epicatechin, four dimeric procyanidins A1, B1, B2, and B4*

Even the alkaloid content of the same species can vary dramatically. Why this occurs is still not well understood. For some species the explanation seems to be that it is caused by climate changes. Concentrations of alkaloids in some species do change as the temperature and climatic conditions change (e.g., wet to dry season).

Even more remarkably, sometimes when two plants are growing side by side, one may be rich in an alkaloid, while a plant of the same species just a few feet away is completely devoid of that same alkaloid. Understanding the significance of this observation is important. Some companies selling Cat's Claw go through unusual measures to analyze the alkaloid content of the plant they plan to harvest *before* removing the plant's bark or root. This adds considerably to the cost of the finished product. Out in the field, only those plants containing the desired range of certain alkaloids are harvested. In the case of companies removing part of the root for harvesting, these extra precautions are important to ensure that the finished product does in fact contain the range of alkaloids that consumers expect.

Some species of *Uncaria* have alkaloids that are unique to them, and are not found in any other species of *Uncaria* in the world, for example as the roxburghines D and X which are unique to *U. elliptica*. Some alkaloids are found only in certain species that grow very far apart. *U. bernaysii* is found only in New Guinea, while *U. guianensis*, is found only in the Amazon region, yet each share the same alkaloid, angustine, which is found in virtually no other species of *Uncaria*.

Heightened interest on the part of the pharmacological industry will probably add to the list of alkaloids discovered in *Uncaria*. Besides the alkaloids, glycosides, tannins, polyphenols, many other compounds also interest scientists, as these too may provide useful therapeutic benefits. This certainly helps us to understand why it is so important to protect the world's forests and botanical habitats. Once a potentially valuable plant is lost due to natural disasters or manmade destruction, its secret store of naturally derived chemicals is almost certain to be lost forever.

ANALYTICAL FINDINGS: WHICH PART OF THE PLANT IS THERAPEUTIC?

The alkaloids found in various species of *Uncaria* are identified by such analytical techniques as: mass spectrometry, capillary zone electrophoresis, liquid chromatography, radioimmunoassay and nuclear magnetic resonance.

In addition to varying in presence from species to species, absent from some and present in some, or perhaps only in one, alkaloid content may also vary in location in different species. For example, the alkaloid angustine is found only in the flowers of *U. bernaysii*; however, in *U. guianensis* it is found in the flowers, the stems and the leaves.

The leaves and stems of *U. tomentosa* contain at least four alkaloids: rhychophylline, isorynchophylline, hirsutine, and dihydrocorynantheine. According to Klaus Keplinger, the leaves have comparable immune stimulating properties as the root, despite the absence of isopteropodine, the alkaloid in *U. tomentosa* that many have attributed as *the* immune potentiator.[14]

Quantitative analysis of the alkaloids of *U. rhynchophylla* found in a number of species of *Uncaria* has repeatedly demonstrated that the composition of the indole and oxindole alkaloids contents varies markedly depending on the species and the part of the plant tested.[15-17] These findings suggest that the biogenetic relationships of the alkaloids in *Uncaria* are not so clearly defined and may require considerably closer examination to determine how they may be related.

While the oxindole alkaloids make up approximately 97% of the total alkaloids in the hook, small stem and leaf of *U. rhynchophylla*, the indole alkaloids are found almost exclusively (approximately 96%) in the bark of the root. The bark of the aerial vine part of *U. rhynchophylla* contains nearly equal parts of the oxindole and indole alkaloids; the alkaloidal content is very low in the (aerial or underground) wood part, while the content of the oxindole and indole alkaloids vary between 2.3% to 8.1%, and 1.8% to 31.1%, respectively, in the wood.

As has been mentioned several times previously, potential sources of the beneficial alkaloids found in *Uncaria* can come from numerous parts of the plant. The dried hooks and stems of most *Uncaria* species have been claimed by traditional healers to possess sedative and antispasmodic actions that can relieve headache and dizziness due to hypertension, and infantile nervous disorders.[18] This may be explained by the presence of the oxindole alkaloids, rhynchophylline and particularly, isohydrocadambine, found in a number of *Uncaria* species that are known to cause an increase in respiratory rate, vasodilation and hypotension.[19-21]

In rats with spontaneous hypertension (high blood pressure) it has been shown that the isodihydrocadambine found in the hooks of *Uncaria* has a dose-dependent hypotensive and antihypertensive effect that is much stronger than even that of another major alkaloid found in many *Uncaria* species, rhynchophylline. The antihypertensive effect has been attributed to isodihydrocadambine's vasodilating activity on peripheral arteries. This would also explain the clinical effectiveness of hooks from *U. rhynchophylla* in the treatment of headache.

The alkaloid mitraphylline is found in several species of *Uncaria*, including *U. attenuata, U. quadrangularis, U. kawakamii, U. elliptica* and *U. tomentosa*. Mitraphylline is a hypotensive agent that acts as a weak central nervous system depressant.[22] The concentration of mitraphylline will vary depending on the part of the plant analyzed. For example, in *U. quadrangularis*, the alkaloids mitraphylline and isomitraphylline are found only in the leaves, while the alkaloids pteropodine and isopteropodine are only found in the stem bark.[23] Therefore, if you are hoping to use *U. quadrangularis* for its hypotensive action, it is important to make sure that the leaves provide the source of the finished product.

A listing of the parts of *Uncaria* that can contain alkaloids is shown in Table 4.

Table 4

PLANT PARTS OF *UNCARIA* SPECIES THAT CAN CONTAIN VARIOUS ALKALOIDS

Apical bud	Basal, old stem
Below apical, young leaf	Bark, inner
Intermediate, mature leaf	Bark, outer
Basal, old leaf	Hook
Below apical, young twig	Root
Intermediate, mature stem	Root bark

The dried hooks and stems of *U. sinesis, U. rhynchophylla, U. macrophylla, U. hirsuta,* and *U. sessilifructus* are used in traditional Chinese medicine and Taiwanese medicine for the treatment of hypertension, headache, epilepsy (in children) and dizziness. They have been attributed to the alkaloids rhynchophylline[24] and isorhynchophylline.[25,26] The modern *Chinese Pharmacopoeia* mentions these alkaloids.[27] Studies have also found that several additional alkaloids, including, dihydrocorynantheine, hirsutine, hirsuteine, dihydrocadambine and isohydrocadambine, produce both hypotensive and vasodilative effects in rats and dogs.[25,28] Yet it is the opinion of many plant pharmacologists that the most important vasodalitive and hypotensive alkaloids found in some species of *Uncaria* are hirsutine, dihyrocorynantheine, and the heteroyohimbines (i.e. gambirdine).

Hirsutine is found in about 11% of the crude base fraction of the extract of the *Uncaria* hooks and stems that contain the hook. It possesses autonomic ganglionic blocking action, antiarrhythmic action, and hypotensive action, in addition to a very mild central depressive action.[29] This may explain why the dried stem segments containing the hooks have been used by practitioners of both traditional Japanese and Chinese medicine as an analgesic, spasmolytic or hypotensive agent. In traditional Chinese medicine, 10 to 15 grams of the stems containing the hooks of *U. hirsuta* are boiled in water for 15 minutes and used for the following conditions: infantile convulsion, high fever, night screaming; colds, headache, neural headache; and hypertension, dizziness, and blurred vision.[30] Hirsutine has been shown to inhibit norephinephrine- and high potassium-induced contractions in the aorta, similar to the action associated with calcium channel blockers (by blockade of calcium influx through voltage-dependent calcium channels).[31] This suggests that "the vasodilative effect of hirsutine is due to inhibition of trans-membrane calcium influx through the voltage-dependent calcium channel."[28] These findings help doctors understand the mechanism of action of the naturally occurring alkaloids in various species of *Uncaria* that contain hirsutine.

Researchers seeking new antihypertensive agents have demonstrated that the heteroyohimbine alkaloid gambirdine found in the Malaysian *Uncaria* species, *U. callophylla*, is also effective in lowering blood pressure. Using gambirdine in rats has resulted in lowering blood pressure. The authors of the rat study concluded that the *Uncaria* species traditionally used in treating hypertension could owe their effect "to the presence of various pharmacologically active antihypertensive alkaloids such as dihyrocorynantheine and gambirdine as well as possibly other yohimbines and heteroyohimbines commonly found in small quantities in such plants."[32]

Rhyncophylline is another important alkaloid found in *U. rhynchophylla* and *U. tomentosa* that has been shown in mice, rats, and rabbits, to have inhibitory effects on platelet aggregation and thrombosis (thromboembolism).[33,34] It has been shown that rhyncophylline is able to suppress malondialdehyde (MDA) formation and platelet factor 4 (PF4) release, thereby suggesting that this specific alkaloid may be a promising antithrombotic agent—i.e., that it may help prevent blood clots in blood vessels.

Other glycosides isolated from *Uncaria* species can also be beneficial. *U. guianensis*, one of the *Uncaria* species found in the Amazonian area of Brazil, and commonly known as "garabato" and "unganangi," and sometimes confused with *U. tomentosa*, has been used by practitioners of traditional Peruvian medicine for the treatment of intestinal ailments, wound healing, arthritis, some cancers and diabetes mellitus, and as a potent anti-inflammatory agent.[35,36] Analytical studies have found that the bark of *U. guianensis* and *U. tomentosa* contains numerous non-alkaloid glycosides, including quinovic acids, that might explain its successful use in traditional medicine.[37] *U. tomentosa* and *U. guianensis* contain very similar glycosides and alkaloids.

A short list of some of the biologically active chemicals found naturally occurring in various species of *Uncaria* is given in Table 5.

Table 5

BIOLOGICALLY ACTIVE CHEMICALS FOUND IN THE GENUS *UNCARIA*[38-40]

Chemical	Biological activity
Beta-sitosterol	anti-inflammatory antialcoholic, antiarthritic, anticariogenic, antihistaminic, antioxidant, antiperiodontal, antiulcer, cancer-preventive
Catechins	
D-catechol	antihepatitic, antiseptic hypotensive, sedative adrenergic blocker, hypotensive anticataract, antiretroviral, antioxidant, antiviral, antitumor, cancer-preventive
Coryantheine	
Dihydrocorynantheine	
Ellagic acid	
Gallic acid	anticarcinomic, antioxidant, antiviral, cancer-preventive
Gambirine	hypotensive
Hirsuteine	hypotensive
Hirsutine	myorelaxant, antihypertensive, hypotensive
Hyperin	anti-inflammatory, antioxidant, diuretic, hepatoprotective
Isorhynchophylline	antihypotensive
Mitraphylline	hypotensive, myorelaxant, vasodilator
Quercetin	antiallergic, antianaphylactic, antiasthmatic, anticataract, antidiabetic, antiviral, antitumor, cancer-preventive
Rhynchophylline	hypotensive, sedative, anti-inflammatory, vasodilator
Rutin	anticataract, antidermatatic, antiviral, antidiabetic, antitumor

PERUVIAN BARKS

The healing properties of various barks that grow on trees, shrubs and vines in Peru, Colombia, and Ecuador, have been known by Europeans since at least 1640.

A 1988 article in the *British Medical Journal* told how Spanish missionaries observed the practices of local Andean healers to learn how they treated a malady known as "marsh fever." Eventually their observation led to the discovery of a secret concoction of Peruvian bark that was used to treat this fever.[41] In 1677 the bark was identified by the Latin name *Cortex peruanus* in the third edition of the *London Pharmakopeia*. In 1742 the Swedish naturalist Linnaeus immortalized the Countess of Chinchon, vice-queen of Peru—who had been cured of a fever by the potent bark and brought a lot of it back to Spain—by misspelling her name as "cinchona" in constructing the generic name for the tree. Soon it was discovered that the bark contained two different alkaloids, quinine and cinchonine, which could be used to treat malaria. The disease—now, but not then, known to be a parasitic infection of the red blood cells by the protozoa of the genus *Plasmodium*—is characterized by attacks of chills, fever and sweating that occur at intervals determined by the time required for the development of a new generation of parasites in the body. The parasite is transmitted by the bites of infected mosquitoes of the genus *Anopheles*, an insect common to many tropical areas of the world.

In the early 19th century it was discovered that the seeds from the cinchona tree had a remarkably high quinine content of around 11 to 13%, compared with the usual yield of less than 3% from other sources. Recognizing the importance of this tree's quinine content, the seeds of the tree were later planted in Java. By 1877, some 20,000 trees were growing on plantations in the Dutch East Indies (now Indonesia), which became the world's major source for this bark. It sold for more money in Amsterdam than any other bark in the world. Eventually the tree became known by its current Latin name, *Cinchona ledgeriana*. When the Japanese occupied the Dutch East Indies during World War II, Allied nations needed a reliable source of quinine. By 1943 the Allies started to give their troops synthetic quinine to meet the need for an antimalarial drug, which led to the decline of the cinchona bark harvesting and processing industry in Indonesia. Subsequent studies of the bark's chemistry led to the discoveries that the bark also contained other alkaloids and that quinine could be converted into quinidine for the treatment of cardiac arrhythmias.

Interestingly, in recent years malarial resistance to the synthetic antimalarial compounds has developed. This has resulted in a revival of interest in quinine and quinidine. With new biotechnology, bioreactors are providing large-scale production of quinine to make up for the lack of adequate supplies of cinchona trees.

But this story gets even more interesting. Quinine, the alkaloid derived from the bark of the cinchona tree, stimulated other discoveries in medicine. The isolation of quinine and other cinchona tree alkaloids in the early part of the 19th century led to the effort to synthesize quinine. While attempting this, the chemist William H. Perkin stumbled upon mauve purple, the first synthetic aniline dye. The use of this dye in microbiology and histopathology made possible major discoveries by other scientists, such as Paul Ehrlich, who discovered the use of aniline dyes to treat malaria and another protozoal infection, trypanosomiasis, which developed into the search for specific antimicrobial agents. This led to the discovery of sulphonamides by Gerhard Domagk in the middle 1930s, and that in turn stimulated the development of antibiotics.

It's a long chain of causation, but all these discoveries were the end results of a secret concoction made by native healers in Peru!

Another plant found in the Amazonian basin of Peru, Ecuador and Colombia is *Maytenus laevis*. This plant has several active substances—phenoldienones (tingenone, 22-hydroxytingenone), a catechin, and two proanthcyanidins—that have antitumor and anti-inflammatory properties. The known biological activities of these compounds confirm the therapeutic claims made by traditional Peruvian healers for extracts of this plant.[42]

Cinchona ledgeriana and *Maytenus laevis* are two examples of the kind of barks found in Peru of interest to medical scientists. Another plant bark (and root) that has attracted considerable interest in recent years comes from the vine *Uncaria tomentosa*. Just what is *Uncaria tomentosa*? How is one to know if it is the genuine item? What is its therapeutic value?

UNCARIA TOMENTOSA (WILD.) DC—"CAT'S CLAW"

History

Cat's Claw has a long history of traditional use in Peruvian and Colombian folk medicine. It is believed that *Uncaria tomentosa* spread from Colombia to Panama and Peru. Some botanists and Peruvian authorities on folk medicine estimate that *U. tomentosa* has been used as a remedy for various ailments for at least several hundred years, especially by many native groups living in eastern Peru, such as the Ashaninka, Cashibo and Campa Indians. Today the Ashaninka Indians are often employed by companies harvesting the plant.

As mentioned earlier, the common name for *Uncaria tomentosa* in Spanish-speaking countries is "Uña de Gato"—Cat's Claw—because of the small, clawlike, downward-pointed hooks at the junction of each stem.

Decoctions of Cat's Claw are used by traditional Peruvian healers for the treatment of arthritis, intestinal infections, wound healing, some cancers and several epidemic diseases.[43,44] The plants grow from southern Mexico through Central America to South America, particularly in the high Amazonian basins of eastern Peru, in the valleys of the Perene and Paucartambo Rivers and in the neighboring highlands.

One of the earliest references to Cat's Claw in the English language dates from 1892, when the botanist Millspaugh explained that the bark from this plant was not to be confused with "Gambier, or pallid catchu, *Uncaria gambier*, Rox."[45] It is interesting to note that *Potter's New Cyclopaedia of Botanical*

Drugs and Preparations, published in 1907, makes no reference to *U. tomentosa,* although it does mention *U. gambier.*

U. tomentosa is sometimes physically confused with another *Uncaria* species, also called "Uña de Gato" and found in Central and South America, *U. guianensis.* Unlike *U. tomentosa* which is found growing in relative abundance at higher elevations of the Peruvian Amazon, around 650 to 2,500 meters above sea level, *U. guianensis* grows at fairly low elevations. This, unfortunately, does not provide as useful a means of distinguishing the two species as one might hope, as *U. tomentosa* has been found growing at quite low elevations throughout most of its range, as well as at high altitudes. For example, the *Annals of the Missouri Botanical Garden* of 1980 illustrates the plant Uña de Gato in its section on the "Flora of Panama." Panama is not known for its mountains! In 1993, researchers associated with the Smithsonian Institution reported finding *U. tomentosa* during a 1990 and 1991 expedition to Barro Colorado Island, Panama, in an area close to sea level.[46] These observations appear to negate the claim by some that the genuine Cat's Claw can come only from higher altitudes in the Andes.

THERAPEUTIC USE

There is considerable controversy among researchers and manufacturers over which part of the plant is therapeutic. Some claim it is the inner bark of the Cat's Claw, others say it doesn't matter as long as it is the bark, and others contend that it's the root. Often it seems that those promoting one part of the plant over another sell only the part of the plant they claim is therapeutic. But what does the literature say?

Researchers at the Institute of Pharmacology at the University of Innsbruck, Austria, have used a patented extract of the root bark called Krallendorn-Kapseln for more than ten years in the treatment of certain types of cancer and several viral diseases.[47] Because of promising results in earlier human trials, the Institute confirmed the existence of six alkaloids in the root bark of *U. tomentosa*: pteropodine, isomitraphylline, uncarine F, mitraphylline, and speciophylline.[48] Some of these alkaloids are described previously in our discussion of various Asian species of *Uncaria*.

Further analytical studies by the Institute resulted in the discovery that a much cruder extract of a commercially available preparation of the root of Cat's Claw yielded virtually the same profile of alkaloids as the pharmaceutical extract.[49] (For you scientists out there who need proof that the crude extract could be almost identical to a pharmaceutical extract, consider that the curves obtained [$r^2=0.999$] were linear in the range of 0.01=1 mg/ml and overlapped [the standard deviation for the six analyses was between 0.5 and 5.2% for all compounds studied], and the detection limit was approximately 0.003 mg for both compounds.) This suggests that the commercially available root powders can have nearly the same profile of alkaloids as the much more expensive pharmaceutical grade extract. However, this depends on the purity of the crude extract and the content of the alkaloids in the Cat's Claw so harvested.

An *in vitro* (test-tube) study by Wagner and colleagues at the Institute of Pharmaceutical Biology at the University of Munich, Germany, isolated the same six alkaloids in their samples of the root of *U. tomentosa* as was reported by the University of Innsbruck.[50] One of these alkaloids, isopteropodine, was found to be "a powerful stimulant of phagocytosis in the range of 10^{-3} -10^{-6} mg/ml."[51] (Phagocytes—the name means "eating cells"—ingest microorganisms or other cells and foreign particles that enter the bloodstream. Phagocytosis is the name for that process of ingestion.) Three other alkaloids, pterodine, isomitraphylline and isorhynchophylline, showed much less phagocytic activity. The other two alkaloids, mitraphylline and rhynchophylline, showed no phagocytic activity. The authors concluded that the observed immunostimulative activity of *U. tomentosa* "may explain the use of various *Uncaria* species for wound-healing, intestinal infections and for the treatment of cancer."

Potentially beneficial nonalkaloid compounds in Cat's Claw have also attracted the interest of researchers. In two studies, nine nonalkaloid glycosides were successfully isolated in the bark of *U. tomentosa*, of which three of the glycosides had never before been found in nature.[47,52] The main steroidic fraction (60%) of Cat's Claw is beta-sitosterol, with lesser amounts of stigmasterol, and campesterol. Preliminary pharmacological investigations have demonstrated that all three steroids, particularly the main sterol, beta-sitosterol, have moderate anti-inflammatory activity.[53]

A study of the potential antiviral activity of an extract of *U. tomentosa* demonstrated that these glycosides do possess moderate antiviral activity *in vitro*[52] against the vesicular stomatitis virus and the rhinovirus type 1B (a flu virus).[66] However, the researchers did admit that the antiviral effect occurred "at relatively high concentrations with respect to the toxic dose . . ." What does this mean? At first appearance, it would appear that in order to get an antiviral effect from such an extract of *U. tomentosa*, one should expect side effects. However, one cannot reach this conclusion so easily. It is entirely possible that the bark contains other compounds which diminish the likelihood of side effects. This may explain why individuals using the crude bark or root of Cat's Claw rather than an extract report less side effects (so far as the scientific literature indicates). It will be interesting to see if people begin to report more side effects once potent standardized extracts of Cat's Claw appear on the market.

Cat's Claw has also been shown to produce anti-inflammatory activity in arthritics. In 1991, researchers studying the glycosides in the root bark of *U. tomentosa* discovered a new quinovic acid glycoside that had never before been seen in nature. It was found that this glycoside had active anti-inflammatory effects.[54] Using a conventional animal model, the researchers determined that this new glycoside was the compound responsible for the anti-inflammatory activity in *U. tomentosa*.

Some promoters of Cat's Claw in the United States and Europe have claimed that it is a cancer preventative and cancer curative. The status of Cat's Claw's value in the prevention or treatment of cancer remains speculative but encouraging.

In vitro studies of the plant extracts and fractions of *U. tomentosa* have shown them to be protective against ultraviolet (UV-A)-induced and chemical-induced (8-methoxypsoralen) mutagenicity.[55] This is an important finding.

In 1993, the first study of the antimutagenic activity of the bark of U. tomentosa in humans was reported by a group of researchers from several universities in Italy. Two individuals were given a decoction of U. tomentosa each day for 15 days (as would be prescribed by a traditional Peruvian healer). One of the subjects was a nonsmoker. The other was a pack-a-day smoker who had smoked for 15 years. Both volunteers were 35 years of age and in overall good health, with no evidence of cancer. The decoction given each subject was obtained by boiling in water 6.5 grams of the dried bark of U. tomentosa for three hours until the initial volume was reduced to about one third, as would be prescribed by a traditional Peruvian healer. Urine samples were taken before and during the study and eight days after the completion of the study. A bacterium was added to the urine samples to test for mutagenicity. This test determines whether there is evidence that genetic mutagenic activity is occurring which could possibly lead to certain types of cancers. The nonsmoker's urine did not show any mutagenic activity before, during or after U. tomentosa treatment. However, the smoker's urine had mutagenic activity before treatment which "showed a dramatic decrease of mutagenic potential at the end of the treatment, persisting until 8 days after the end of the treatment."[55,pp.74-75] No other studies confirming these findings have so far been reported.

The antimutagenic effect of Cat's Claw as discussed above *in vitro* and *in vivo* leads us to wonder how it is that U. tomentosa can be a cancer-preventative agent. The Italian researchers speculate that the significant antimutagenic activity of the U. tomentosa extracts and fractions may be due to antioxidant action. The Italians conducted an *in vitro* study that found that U. tomentosa can quench singlet oxygen which scavenges other oxygen radicals, thereby acting as a classic antioxidant. In the case of the smoker, the investigators believed the inhibitory effect of U. tomentosa "may be due to an antioxidant mechanism which acts by inhibiting oxidative/free radical mediators in the transformation of the procarcinogens present in cigarette smoke to ultimate carcinogens."[55,p.76] This is the first clear evidence that *U. tomentosa* may be a possible cancer preventative. Obviously, much more research is needed before we can do much more than speculate.

Further support for this idea comes from a 1993 study in which, investigators were able to determine that the alkaloid uncarine F was able to inhibit proliferation of leukemic cells (cell lines HL 60 and U-9), while at the same concentration not inhibiting progenitor cells obtained from normal human bone marrow.[56] The investigators concluded that "uncarine F may be considered as a possible drug for the treatment of patients with acute leukemia," thereby suggesting that uncarine F in *U. tomentosa* is the most likely candidate for inhibiting the proliferation of leukemic cells in humans. This does *not* mean, however, that *U. tomentosa* has been shown to be an effective treatment agent in human leukemia. Further studies demonstrating this effect are needed.

With the exception of two alkaloids, mitraphylline and rhynchophylline, all alkaloids in an extract of *U. tomentosa* have been shown to cause a pronounced enhancement of phagocytosis, *in vitro* and *in vivo*.[50]

Method of Use

The recommended initial intake of *U. tomentosa* is two to five 150-milligram capsules a day on an empty stomach. Individuals experiencing gastrointestinal disturbance following the ingestion of the capsules should consider removing the contents of the capsules and mixing it in a cup of cold water. Slowly heat the water in a small pan for about ten minutes until it boils. Wait until the tea has cooled down before drinking. The taste will be bitter. Consume 3 to 4 cups per day if drinking a tea. If using a liquid extract, restrict use to 15–25 days, 3–4 times per day.

Whenever a "decoction" of Cat's Claw is recommended, mix the fine powder with cold water and allow the mixture to simmer on a stove for 45 minutes at a temperature of 80° Celsius (176° Fahrenheit). Decoctions are generally made in a strength of 30 grams (around one ounce) of powder to

800-850 milliliters (approximately one and one-half pints) of water to leave around 500 ml of simmered-down liquid. When cool, the decoction is strained through filter paper and taken in the recommended divided doses. Like infusions, decoctions should be prepared fresh every day and kept in a tightly sealed bottle at room temperature. The adult dose is approximately 60 ml (two ounces) of the decoction mixed with 60 ml of hot water on an empty stomach in the morning. For children ages three to six, the dosage should be 20 ml of the tea with 20 ml of hot water in the morning. For older children, adjust accordingly.

ANALYTICAL PROFILE FOR THE DETERMINATION OF *UNCARIA TOMENTOSA*

U. guianensis, the only other *Uncaria* species that has been identified in the Amazon region, has often been confused with *U. tomentosa*. One fairly obvious reason is that people in and around Peru and other pantropical regions of Latin America have unfortunately used the Spanish name "uña de gato" to describe both species. It helps, but not enough, that *U. guianensis* is locally known also as "uña de gavilan" and "garabato" in Spanish. The continuing confusion is one reason it is important to buy Cat's Claw from a reliable source. Many of the compounds found in *U. tomentosa* (listed in Table 6) are not found in *U. guianensis*, allowing an easy way to distinguish between the two species. *U. guianensis* does not contain the alkaloids isopteropodine, speciophylline, uncarine F, rotundifoline and isorotundifoline (see Table 3). While pteropodine and isopteropodine are richest in the root and bark of *U. tomentosa*, it is the mitraphyllines, mitraphylline and isomitraphylline, that are the major alkaloids in *U. guianensis*. Usually it is adequate to check for the presence of the alkaloids isopteropodine, speciophylline, isorotundifoline and rotundifoline to be sure that the product is genuine *Uncaria tomentosa*. Further guidelines on confirming the analytical profile of genuine Cat's Claw are provided later.

Table 6

COMPOUNDS IDENTIFIED IN *U. TOMENTOSA*

Alkaloids:

Carboxystrictosidine	Isorhynchophylline
Dihydrocorynantheine	Mitraphylline
Hirsuteine	Pteropodine
Hirsutine	Rotundifoline
Isomitraphylline	Rynchophylline
Isopteropodine	Speciophylline
Isorotundifoline	Uncarine F

Steroids:

Beta-sitosterol	Campesterol
Stigmasterol	

Polyhydroxylated triterpenes

Three major glycosides

Six quinovic acid glycosides (a 7th only in the root)

Only a few laboratories in the United States and Europe have sufficient experience or adequate equipment to analyze *U. tomentosa* according to the most modern methods of analysis. Two laboratories that have considerable experience analyzing *U. tomentosa* and other *Uncaria* species are the Institute of Pharmacognosy at the University of Innsbruck, Austria and, Immodal Pharmaka GmbH in Volders, Austria.

In 1994, Immodal Pharmaka published a paper showing that different varieties of the freshly cut root of *U. tomentosa* (white-gray, yellow-brown, and dark red root bark) contained varying levels of the six major alkaloids. Two alkaloids in *U. tomentosa*, rhynchophylline and isorhynchophylline, were present at significantly higher levels in the yellow-brown variety of the root than in either of the other two root varieties. For all samples studied by the same laboratory over a period of several years, individual plants were found to have "switched from one alkaloid pattern to the other over the years [yet] in all instances either the pteropodine and mitraphylline isomers or the rhynchophyllines were found as major constituents. The total alkaloid content varied from 0.036 to 3.83% (wet weight) of dried root bark."[57] This report is important because it helps to explain the inconsistent findings on the percentage of the alkaloid content of various samples of U. *tomentosa* reported by earlier researchers and variations among lots of the product.

ECOLOGICAL ISSUES

In a paper on the chemical investigation of the alkaloid contents of tropical plants, Dr. David Phillipson of the University of London claims that nothing is known about the chemical composition of over 99% of the Brazilian flora. He fears that the next century may be characterized by an enormous rate of extinction of these plants.[58]

The frightening thought has emerged that it is doubtful whether 5% of the world's organisms can be investigated chemically before the remaining 80% become extinct. This has led to the view that if no register is made of the molecules perfected by nature over 3 billion years of evolution then not only are we destroying a powerful telescope for looking into our past but we are endangering our future.

TOXICOLOGY

Cat's Claw, in whatever form, should not be taken by women who are planning on becoming pregnant in the near future, are pregnant, or are breast-feeding. Anyone who has recently had or is scheduled to receive a organ transplant or skin-graft should not take Cat's Claw. *U. tomentosa* can cause the immune system to reject transplanted cells.

Some herbalists are reluctant to recommend a high dose of a decoction of *U. tomentosa* because of concerns that it contains too much catechu (*(+)-catechinin*), a catechol tannin. Catechu is a potentially toxic astringent when used excessively in the treatment of diarrhea. However, catechu is found in *U. gambir*, not *U. tomentosa*. Excessive intake of tannins in the diet is recognized as a dietary carcinogen and antinutrient interfering with the body's full use of protein. Nevertheless, caution is advised, since it is estimated that the bark of *U. tomentosa* contains up to 20% tannins.

U. tomentosa contains rhynchophylline. The LD_{50} (lethal dose for half the litter) in mice for this alkaloid, is 162 milligrams per kilogram of body weight. It is highly unlikely that anyone could ever consume enough *U. tomentosa* to cause an acute episode of rhynchophylline toxicity. Nevertheless, it is not known if subacute toxicity would occur due to long-term use. In mice, the water extract of the root of *U. tomentosa* when taken orally did not produce any toxicity when five grams per kilogram of body weight were given.[14]

Kallendorn, a standardized extract of *U. tomentosa* sold in some European countries, has been studied for its acute and subacute toxicity. Based on these studies the following contraindications are recommended for those using Kallendorn Cat's Claw:

1) Pregnant and nursing women should not use the product, due to lack of adequate safety studies.
2) Children under age 3 should not take the product, for the same reason.
3) Do not use the product when bone marrow transplants are expected in cases of leukemia—at least one year should pass following the use of the product before a transplant should be considered.
4) Do not use if any organ transplant operation is planned.
5) The product is contraindicated in cases of deliberate drug-induced immune suppression.

In cases where *U. tomentosa* is used in the treatment of autoimmune diseases or tumors, up to two weeks of constipation, diarrhea or fever may occur. This can sometimes be avoided by reducing the dosage, or discontinuing use for three days before and after treatment.

The manufacturers of Kallendorn recommend that all extracts of *U. tomentosa* be discontinued two days before and two days after chemotherapy because of its strong immunostimulating effect. This also applies to treatments utilizing foreign proteins, such as hormone therapies using animal proteins, passive immunization and thymus therapy. There is no problem with its use with active immunization, according to the manufacturer, although it should not be taken in combination with hyperimmunoglobulin therapy.

We have seen that *Uncaria guianensis* has been mistakenly called Cat's Claw in some parts of South America, but there is a more dangerous possibility of confusion closer to home. A September 5, 1995 article in the *Corpus Christi* [Texas] *Caller-Times* reported that some members of the local Hispanic community were buying Cat's Claw at local flea markets and in some local stores.[59] Unfortunately, some of the products were mislabeled and found to be *Acacia greggii*, a common shrub that grows along the United States and Mexican border. This shrub contains a chemical compound that contains cyanide and is not fit for human consumption. This incident underscores the need for Cat's Claw to be correctly identified not only by its Latin name, but also by reliable independent analyses. Buy Cat's Claw from a reputable source that stands behind its analysis and labeling. For this reason, I have provided the following information on obtaining genuine *U. tomentosa*.

HOW TO BE SURE IT'S GENUINE CAT'S CLAW

There are a number of companies in the United States offering Cat's Claw products. Those listed below responded to my request for further information about their products and samples for analysis. Each company listed is also a member of the National Natural Products Association (NNFA), of Newport Beach, California. The NNFA requires all manufacturers who wish to be members to agree to submit all of their labels to the Tru-Label program. The program randomly analyzes products sold in the natural products industry. Companies selling herbs should also be members of the American Herbal Products Association (AHPA). Members of AHPA adhere to standards of trade that are designed to protect consumers from mislabeled herbs.

Let me dispel a rumor that I had heard from several sources. Rumors that it is illegal to harvest the root of *U. tomentosa* in Peru are false, and are exploded by information supplied by the Peruvian Ministry of Agriculture. What *is* illegal is the commercial export of live plants from Peru.

Further, it is not true that the only source of Cat's Claw is Peru, as some suppliers have claimed. *U. tomentosa* is found in southern Mexico, all of Central America, and in most of the countries within the tropical and sub-tropical belt of South America, including Ecuador, Colombia, Venezuela and Peru. The total alkaloid content of *U. tomentosa* from various sources outside of Peru remains unknown.

Also, claims that a company is selling only the "inner bark" are without foundation. Field observations made in Peru on behalf of this author by local residents found that much of the whole bark is ground into a fine powder, not just the few millimeters of the inner bark. One company is trying to get a true inner bark powder on the market, but could not supply this author with the name of any brand. Although it is true that in most cases the inner bark does contains higher concentration of the three referenced alkaloids of *U. tomentosa* (isopteropodine, pteropodine and uncarine F), the whole bark should also contain these three alkaloids. It is important that there be at least 0.30 to 0.90 grams per 100 grams respectively of the alkaloids isopteropodine, pteropodine and uncarine F. Consumers should insist on an independent certificate of analysis showing that the product being sold is within this range, or that the total alkaloid content, including these three specific alkaloids, is between 0.30 to 1.30 grams per 100 grams. The lot number of the product being sold should correspond with the lot number analyzed.

An example of an independent HPLC laboratory analysis of genuine Cat's Claw *root* is shown in Table 7.

A HPLC laboratory analysis performed by an Austrian labo-

Table 7

HPLC ANALYSIS OF CAT'S CLAW ROOT

Compound	Sample (Lot #)	g/100g	Relative %
Pteropodine	0.2338++/-	0.0100	38.00
Isopteropodine	0.1630++/-	0.0040	27.00
Uncarine F	0.0301++/-	0.0009	5.00
Mitraphylline	0.0570++/-	0.0012	9.00
Compound	Sample (Lot #)	g/100g	Relative %
Isomitraphylline	0.0451++/-	0.0029	7.00
Rhynchopylline	0.0391++/-	0.0018	6.00
Isorhynchopylline	0.0444++/-	0.0015	7.00
Speciophylline	0.0330++/-	0.0015	5.00
TOTAL	0.6100		100.00

ratory on a Cat's Claw root product sold as Vida Vital by Immuno Vital Inc. of Miami, Florida revealed the alkaloid profile shown in Table 8. The analysis was received by this author on December 9, 1995, for Lot #62095. This profile confirms the alkaloid profile associated with genuine Cat's Claw root. It is particularly rich in the indole alkaloids associated with *U. tomentosa*, probably owing to selective harvesting.

Samples of three commercially available Cat's Claw bark capsules containing "500 mg. of Cat's Claw bark" submitted for analysis to an Austrian laboratory found between 40% to 70% less total alkaloid content in the bark than in the root sample in Table 8. The range of total alkaloid content in the bark varied from 0.19 to 0.25, compared to 0.60 to 0.85 for the root.

Concentrated extracts of Cat's Claw may produce side effects and should be treated as classical drugs. Nobody has determined what the ideal concentration range of the alkaloids should be for *U. tomentosa*. However, native healers have used the root and bark for hundreds of years without using an extract. They did not use "standardized extracts" in their traditional practices. Peruvian healers this author consulted with did not have an opinion as to what alkaloids should be used to standardize an extract. In fact they did not care. Their major concern was that the bark or root be genuine Cat's Claw and that the decoctions be prepared according to traditional customs.

Table 8

HPLC ANALYSIS OF COMMERCIAL CAT'S CLAW ROOT

Compound	Sample (Lot #)	g/100g	Relative %
Pteropodine	0.2435++/-	0.0111	39.50
Isopteropodine	0.1625++/-	0.0039	26.36
Uncarine F	0.0264++/-	0.0009	4.29
Mitraphylline	0.0507++/-	0.0010	8.23
Isomitraphylline	0.0368++/-	0.0031	5.98
Rhynchopylline	0.0376++/-	0.0020	6.10
Isorhynchophylline	0.0348++/-	0.0013	5.65
Speciophylline	0.0241++/-	0.0014	3.90
TOTAL	0.6164		100.00

Any effort to introduce a standardized extract of Cat's Claw into the marketplace should be justified by evidence of its clinical efficacy and concomitant lack of toxicity.

Reported toxicity studies of extracts are limited to those done on the product called Kallendorn sold by Immodal Pharmaka in Austria. This extract has been studied for toxicity, and studies of its clinical efficacy for various immune disorders continue. This extract may not fall within the definition of a "dietary supplement" as defined by regulations of the U.S. Food and Drug Administration, under the Dietary Supplement Health and Education Act of 1994. In the interim, it is important to remember that it is the natural bark or root of *U. tomentosa* that has been used by traditional healers for hundreds of years, not an extract.

The sources of genuine Cat's Claw listed below can be warranted as of January, 1996. The reader is encouraged to demand independent laboratory analysis of these suppliers and others selling Cat's Claw for the "lot #" being purchased.

SOURCES OF GENUINE CAT'S CLAW

Immuno Vital, Inc.
2828 Coral Way, Suite 305, Miami, FL 33145
(P.O. Box 450097, Miami, FL 33245)
Phone: 1-800-335-8432; FAX (305) 447-0816

Vida Vital™ by Immuno Vital is the brand name for

Cat's Claw root capsules. 150 mg per capsule. Available in GNC stores and other health food stores.)

Amazon Herb Co.
725 N. A1A, Suite C-115, Jupiter, FL 33477
Phone: 1-800-835-0850; (407) 575-7663; Fax (407) 575-7935
Uña de Gato by Amazon Herb Co. is the brand name for Cat's Claw bark, 500 mg. per capsule. Available in health food stores.

Peruvian Rainforest Botanicals,
Division of Peruvian Imports Unlimited, Inc.
212 N. U.S. Highway One, Suite 17, Tequesta, FL 33469
Phone: 1-800-742-2529; (407) 745-2917; Fax (407) 745-3017
Cat's Claw by Peruvian Rainforest Botanicals is the brand name for Cat's Claw bark, 500 mg. per capsule. Available in health food stores.

For the extract Krallendorn®-Medikamente, contact:
Immodal Pharmaka GmbH,
Bundesstrasse 44, A-6111 Volders, Tirol, Austria
Phone: in Austria (Use "(0)" only within the country):
(0) 52-24-57678; Fax (0) 52-24-57646
It is important to know that owing to U.S. FDA regulations, this product may be classed as a drug, not a dietary supplement, under the definition of the Dietary Supplement Health and Education Act of 1994.

Immuno Vital supplies Cat's Claw root. According to the company it harvests the roots of *U. tomentosa* under a permit "in coordination and compliance with the Reforestry Division of the Peruvian Agriculture Ministry." The root acts like many weeds we are familiar with. Unless all of the root is removed, the remaining root parts will send out new root shoots. The president of Immuno Vital claimed that for every plant harvested two plants are replanted in the same vicinity. Further, his company instructs those commissioned to harvest the root always to leave a portion of the root system intact to assure that the plant can send up a new liana (vine). Before the root is harvested the company has a sample of each potential root stock analyzed for alkaloid content. Only those roots that meet a minimum alkaloid content are considered for harvesting. The others are covered up and left alone.

I find this extra effort encouraging. It is in the tradition established by Charles Ledger in his exploitation of the cinchona trees of Peru, source of the antimalarial alkaloid quinine. Ledger was a British subject who settled in Peru in the 19th century to trade in local goods with various parts of the British Empire. The "quinquina bark trade" attracted him, but the problem was that the trade was hampered by the fact that there were a great variety of cinchona trees, each having a different concentration of alkaloids in its bark. To make sure that his customers had the very best species, *Cinchona calisaya*, he learned everything he could about these trees. His expertise came from local "cascarilleros," the Indians who collected quinquina bark. With the services of those he hired to harvest the best trees he became adept at selecting only the best bark. His field observations led him to learn that the most beautiful cinchona trees were usually the least suitable for exploitation. His concern for harvesting led to people seeking his bark out as the best source of quinquina bark in the world. Although price is an important factor in the competitive natural products market, ultimately it will be up to the consumer to decide if price or *quality* is most important.

Like the Countess of Chinchon, Ledger gained a measure of immortality; the most important species of the tree is now called *Cinchona ledgeriana*.

THANKS

Special thanks are given to: Assistant Professor Else Alschuler, N.D., Assistant Professor of Botanical Medicine, Southwest College of Naturopathic Medicine and Health Sciences, Tempe, Arizona; Allison Blake, Scottsdale, Arizona; Gaia Herbal Educational Services, Cambridge, Massachusetts; the Herb Research Foundation, Boulder, Colorado; the American Botanical Council, Austin, Texas; and those many pioneers who persisted in studying the medicinal potential of *Uncaria Tomentosa*.

REFERENCES

1. Anonymous, Milagro en la Selva: La Uña de Gato. A Miracle of the Peruvian Jungle. *Salud y Naturaleza* (Health and Nature) (date unknown): p. 20-21.
2. Craker, L.E. and J.E. Simon, eds. *Herbs, Spices, and Medicinal Plants: Recent Advances in Botany, Horticulture, and Pharmacology.* Volume 4. 1989, Oryx Press: Phoenix, Ariz. 72, 84.
3. Bensky, D. and A. Gamble, *Chinese Herbal Medicine Materia Medica.* 1986, Seattle: Eastland Press. 603.
4. Hsu, H. et al., *Oriental Materia Medica: A Concise Guide.* 1986, Long Beach, Cal.: Oriental Healing Arts Institute.
5. Hsu, H. and W.G. Peacher, eds. *Chinese Herb Medicine and Therapy.* 1994, Keats Publishing: New Canaan, Conn. 205.
6. Kan, W.S., *Manual of Vegetable Drugs in Taiwan.* Part 2. 1973, Taipei, Taiwan, R.O.C. (Chinese): Chinese Medicine Publishing, 22-23.
7. Lin, C.C. and W.S. Kan, Medicinal plants used for the treatment of hepatitis in Taiwan. *American Journal of Chinese Medicine,* 1990. 18: p. 35-43.
8. Lin, C.C., J.M. Lin, and H.F. Chiu, Studies on folk medicine "thang-kau-tin" from Taiwan. (I). The anti-inflammatory and liver-protective effect. *American Journal of Chinese Medicine,* 1992. 20(1): p. 37-50.
9. Lin, J. et al., Studies on Taiwan folk medicine, Thang-kau-tin (II): Measurement of active oxygen scavenging activity using an ESR technique. *American Journal of Chinese Medicine,* 1995. 23(1): p. 43-51.
10. Gimlette, J.D. and I.J. Burkill, The medicinal book of Malayan Medicine. *Gardens Bulletin Singapore,* 1930. 6: p. 333-439.
11. Anderson, E.F., *Plants and People of the Golden Triangle: Ethnobotany of the Hill Tribes of Northern Thailand.* 1993, Chiang Mai, Thailand: Silkworm Books. 223.
12. Ostendorf, F.W., Nuttige planten en sierplanten in Suriname. *Landbouw Proefstation in Suriname Bulletin,* 1962. 79: p. 199-200.
13. Aimi, N. et al., Studies on plants containing indole alkaloids. VI. Minor bases of Uncaria rhynchophylla Miq. *Chem. Pharm. Bull.,* 1977. 8(25): p. 2067-2071.
14. Keplinger, K. and D. Keplinger, Oxindole alkaloids having properties

stimulating the immunologic system and preparation containing the same, in *United States Patent*. 1994, Keplinger, K.: USA.

15. Lin, C.C. and W.S. Kan, Medicinal plants used for the treatment of hepatitis in Taiwan. *American Journal of Chinese Medicine*, 1990. 18: p. 35-43.

16. Yamanaka, E. et al., Studies of plants containing indole alkaloids. IX. Quantitative analysis on the tertiary alkaloids in various parts of Uncaria rhynchophylla Miq. Yakugaku Zasshi 1983. 103: p. 1028-1033.

17. Nozoye, T., Uncaria alkaloids. XVII. Structure of rhynchophylline. 4. Structure of the side chain in rhynchophylline. *Annual Report of Itsuu Laboratory*, 1957. 8: p. 10-11.

18. Aisaka, K. et al., Hypotensive action of 3-alpha-dihydrocadambine, an indole alkaloid glycoside of Uncaria hooks. *Planta Medica*, 1985: p. 424-427.

19. Akamatsu, M. and T. Kunita, *Nagasaki Medical Journal*, 1928. 6: p. 333.

20. Hori, N., *Nagasaki Medical Journal*. 1931. 9: p. 710.

21. Usui, K., *Shinshu Medical Journal*. 1959. 8: p. 1458.

23. Tantivatana, P. et al., Alkaloids from Uncaria Quadrangularis. *Journal of Medicinal Plant Research*, 1979. 35: p. 92-96.

24. Kondo, H., T. Fukuda, and M. Tomita, Alkaloids of Ouronparia rhynchophylla Matsum. *Journal of the Pharmacology Society of Japan*, 1928. 48: p. 321-337.

25. Endo, K. et al., Hypotensive principles of Uncaria hooks. *Journal of Medicinal Plant Research*, 1983. 49: p. 188-190.

26. Aimi, N., *Traditional Sino-Japan Medicine*, 1987. 8: p. 53-58.

27. Tang, W. and G. Eisenbrand, *Chinese Drugs of Plant Origin: Chemistry, Pharmacology, and Use in Traditional and Modern Medicine*. 1992, Berlin: Springer-Verlag. 997.

28. Yano, S. et al., CA2+ channel blocking effects of hirsutine, an indole alkaloid from Uncaria Genus, in the isolated rat aorta. *Planta Medicina*. 1991. 57: p. 403-405.

29. Kawazoe, S. et al., Method of harvesting the crude drug based on distribution of alkaloids in the hook and in the stem with hook of Uncaria rhynchophylla., in *Planta Medicina*. 1991. p. 47-49.

30. Siu-Cheong, C. and L. Ning-hon, eds. *Chinese Medicinal Herbs of Hong Kong*, Volume 3. Vol. 3. 1993: Hong Kong. 164-165.

31. Horie, S. et al., Effects of hirsutine, an antihypertensive indole alkaloid

from Uncaria rhynchophylla, on intracellular calcium in rat thoracic aorta. *Life Sciences*, 1992. 50(7): p. 491-498.

32. Mok, J.S.L. et al., Cardiovascular responses in the normotensive rat produced by intravenous injection of gambirine isolated from Uncaria callophylla Bl. ex Korth. *Journal of Ethnopharmacology*, 1992. 36: p. 219-223.

33. Jin, R.M. et al., Effect of rhynchophylline on platelet aggregation and experimental thrombosis. *Acta Pharmacologica Sinica*, 1991. 26: p. 246-249.

34. Chang-Xun, C. et al., Inhibitory effect of rhynchophylline on platelet aggregration and thrombosis. *Acta Pharmacologica Sinica*, 1992. 13(2): p. 126-130.

35. Hemingway, S.R. and J.D. Phillipson, Alkaloids from S. American species of Uncaria (Rubiaceae). *Journal of Pharmacology and Pharmaceuticals*, 1974. 26 (Suppl.): p. 113.

36. Yepez, A.M. et al., Quinovic acid glycosides from Uncaria guianensis, in *Phytochemistry*. 1991. p. 1635-1637.

37. Lavault, M., C. Moretti, and J. Bruneton, Alcaloides de I'Uncaria guianensis. *Journal of Medicinal Plant Research*, 1983. 47: p. 244-245.

38. Duke, J.A., *CRC Handbook of Biologically Active Phytochemicals and Their Bioactivities*. 1992, Boca Raton, Fla.: CRC Press.

39. Duke, J.A., *CRC Handbook of Phytochemical Constituents in GRAS Herbs*. 1992, Boca Raton, Fla.: CRC Press.

40. Duke, J.A., Una De Gato. *Business of Herbs*, 1994. 1(2).

41. Bruce-Chwatt, L.J., Three hundred and fifty years of the Peruvian fever bark. *British Medical Journal*, 1988. 296: p. 1485-1486.

42. Gonzalez, J.G. et al., Chuchuhuasha—a drug used in folk medicine in the Amazonian and Andean areas. A chemical study of Maytenus laevis. *Journal of Ethnopharmcology*, 1982. 5(1): p. 73-77.

43. Stuppner, H. et al., A differential sensitivity of oxindole alkaloids to normal and leukemic cell lines. *Planta Medicina*, 1993. Supplement Issue(Supplement Issue): p. A583.

44. Personal communication, 1995.

45. Millspaugh, C.F., *Medicinal Plants*. 1892, Philadelphia: John C. Yorston & Company. 76.

46. Zotz, G. and K. Winter, Short-term photosynthesis measurements predict leafcarbon balance in tropical rain-forest canopy plants, in *Planta*. 1993.

47. Cerri, R. et al., New quinovic acid glycosides from *Uncaria tomentosa*. *Journal of Natural Products*, 1988. 51(2): p. 257-261.
48. Stuppner, H. and S. Sturm, Capillary electrophoretic analysis of oxindole alkaloids from *Uncaria tomentosa*. *Journal of Chromatography*, 1992(June): p. 375-380.
49. Stuppner, H., S. Sturm, and G. Konwalinka, HFLC analysis of the main oxindole alkaloids from *Uncaria tomentosa*. *Chromatography*, 1992. 31(11/12): p. 597-600.
50. Wagner, H., B. Kreutzkamp, and K. Jurcic, Die alkaloid von Uncaria tomentosa und ihre phagozytose-steigernde wirkung. (The alkaloids of Uncaria tomentosa and their phagocytosis-enhancing effect). *Planta Medica*, 1985. 47: p. 419-423.
51. Wagner, H. Immunostimulants from higher plants (recent advances). In *Proceedings of the Phytochemical Society of Europe*. 1987. Oxford: Clarendon Press.
52. Aquino, R., F. De Simone, and C. Pizza, Plant metabolites. Structure and in vitro antiviral activity of quinovic acid glycosides from *Uncaria tomentosa* and *Guettarda platypoda*. *Journal of Natural Products*, 1989. 52(4): p. 679-685.
53. Senatore, A. et al., Phytochemical and biological study of *Uncaria tomentosa* Bollettino—*Societa Italiana Biologia Sperimentale*, 1989. 65(6): p. 517-520.
54. Aquino, R. et al., Plant metabolites. New compounds and antiinflammatory activity of *Uncaria tomentosa*. *Journal of Natural Products*, 1991. 54(2): p. 453-459.
55. Rizzi, R. et al., Mutagenic and antimutagenic activities of *Uncaria tomentosa* and its extracts. *Journal of Ethnopharmacology*, 1993. 38: p. 63-77.
56. Stuppner, H. et al., A differential sensitivity of oxindole alkaloids to normal and leukemic cell lines. *Planta Medicina*, 1993. Supplement Issue (Supplement Issue): p. A583.
57. Laus, G. and D. Keplinger, Separation of steroisomeric oxindole alkaloids from *Uncaria tomentosa* by high performance liquid chromatography. *Journal of Chromotography*, 1994. 662: p. 243-249.
58. Phillipson, J., Chemical investigations of herbarium material for alkaloids. *Journal of Pharmacognosy*, 1982(10): p. 2441-2456.
59. Press, A., Popular herb thought to be poisonous, *Austin* (Texas) *Statesman*. 5 Sept. 1995, p. B3.